THE PREGNANCY DIET BOOK

A Wholesome Guide to a Healthy Pregnancy Diet

DEBORAH W VINSON

Copyright © 2024 [Deborah W Vinson]

All rights reserved. No part of this publication may be reproduced, distributed, or transmitted in any form or by any means, including photocopying, recording, or other electronic or mechanical methods, without the prior written permission of the publisher, except in the case of brief quotations embodied in critical reviews and certain other noncommercial uses permitted by copyright law.

This book is intended for informational purposes only and is not a substitute for professional medical advice, diagnosis, or treatment. Always seek the advice of your physician or other qualified health provider with any questions you may have regarding a medical condition. Never disregard professional medical advice or delay in seeking it because of something you have read in this book.

The publisher and author have made every effort to ensure the accuracy of the information herein. However, the information provided in this book is sold without warranty, either express or implied. The author and publisher will not be held liable for any damages, direct or indirect, arising from the use of the information contained in this book.

TABLE OF CONTENT

1. Introduction
2. Eating for Two: Basics of a Healthy Pregnancy Diet
3. Essential Nutrients for Mom and Baby
4. Building Blocks: Proteins and Their Importance
5. Power of Greens: Incorporating Vegetables
6. Fruits for a Sweet and Nutrient-Rich Pregnancy
7. Grains and Whole Foods: Fueling Your Pregnancy
8. Healthy Fats for Brain Development
9. Hydration: The Key to a Well-Nourished Pregnancy
10. Managing Cravings and Snacking Smartly
11. Meal Planning Made Easy
12. Special Considerations: Allergies, Restrictions, and More

13. Staying Active for a Healthy Pregnancy
14. Postpartum Nutrition: Nourishing Your Body After Birth
15. Recipes for a Vibrant Pregnancy
16. Frequently Asked Questions
17. Conclusion: Embracing a Nutrient-Packed Pregnancy Journey

CHAPTER 1
Introduction

In a world saturated with information and advice on pregnancy, navigating the journey to motherhood can be both exhilarating and overwhelming. As expectant mothers embark on this transformative path, they are bombarded with an avalanche of recommendations, opinions, and guidelines. Amidst this cacophony, the need for a reliable and comprehensive resource becomes paramount. Enter the Pregnancy Diet Book – a beacon of wisdom and nourishment for mothers-to-be, meticulously crafted to guide them through the intricate dance of nutrition during this crucial phase of life.

This groundbreaking tome transcends the ordinary; it is not just a compilation of recipes but a holistic approach to maternal well-being. Authored by leading experts in the fields of nutrition and obstetrics, the Pregnancy Diet Book is more than a guide; it is a companion, a confidante, and a roadmap to optimal health for both mother and baby.

The book unfolds with a profound exploration of the physiological marvel that is pregnancy, demystifying the intricate interplay between a mother's body and the developing life within. It delves into the nuanced changes that occur during each trimester, offering invaluable insights into the nutritional requirements unique to every stage. By intertwining the science of gestation with accessible language, the Pregnancy Diet

Book empowers expectant mothers to make informed choices that resonate with their individual needs.

Central to the book's philosophy is the understanding that pregnancy is not a one-size-fits-all journey. It acknowledges the diversity of maternal experiences, catering to a spectrum of dietary preferences, cultural nuances, and health considerations. Whether a mother adheres to a vegetarian, vegan, or omnivorous diet, the Pregnancy Diet Book provides tailored guidance, ensuring that nutritional needs are met without compromising personal beliefs or values.

The heartbeat of the Pregnancy Diet Book is its meticulously curated recipes – a symphony of flavors designed to satiate cravings, nurture the body, and support the baby's development. From nutrient-packed smoothies that soothe morning sickness to wholesome, hearty meals that fuel energy, the recipes are a gastronomic celebration of the incredible journey of pregnancy. Each dish is a fusion of taste and nutrition, a testament to the idea that nourishment can be both delectable and healthful.

Beyond the culinary realm, the book navigates the often-overlooked terrain of emotional well-being during pregnancy. It addresses the psychological facets of cravings, mood swings, and the emotional rollercoaster that accompanies the miraculous process of bringing life into the world. The Pregnancy Diet Book advocates a holistic approach that recognizes the intricate dance between mind and body, offering strategies for maintaining mental equilibrium amidst the whirlwind of hormonal changes.

In a society where misinformation often eclipses genuine guidance, the Pregnancy Diet Book stands as a beacon of evidence-based knowledge. Backed by the latest research in obstetrics and nutrition, the book dispels myths and misconceptions that may cloud the path to a healthy pregnancy. It empowers mothers with the knowledge to make choices aligned with the latest scientific understanding, fostering a sense of confidence and assurance as they navigate this transformative journey.

Moreover, the Pregnancy Diet Book extends its reach beyond the gestational period, emphasizing the importance of postpartum nutrition and recovery. It recognizes that the journey does not end with childbirth but rather evolves into a new phase of nurturing – both for the mother and her newborn. With practical guidance on postpartum nutrition, the book ensures a seamless transition into the challenges and joys of motherhood.

As a testament to its credibility, the Pregnancy Diet Book is not merely a collection of theoretical ideals. It draws strength from real-life testimonials, weaving the narratives of women who have traversed the path of pregnancy guided by its principles. These stories serve as inspiration and solidarity, creating a community of mothers united by a commitment to optimal health for themselves and their infants.

In essence, the Pregnancy Diet Book is not just a manual; it is a legacy. It is a profound exploration of the sacred journey of pregnancy, a celebration of life's most miraculous moments, and a guiding light for mothers who seek to navigate this transformative passage with grace, knowledge, and nourishment. As it graces the shelves of expectant mothers around the world, it leaves an indelible mark on the landscape of maternal care –

a testament to the power of informed choices, wholesome nutrition, and the enduring spirit of motherhood.

CHAPTER 2
Eating for Two: Basics of a Healthy Pregnancy Diet

Maintaining a healthy diet during pregnancy is crucial for both the mother's well-being and the proper development of the baby. Let's explore the basics of a nutritious pregnancy diet to ensure a smooth journey for both.

1. Nutrient-Rich Foods:
Focus on consuming nutrient-dense foods like fruits, vegetables, whole grains, lean proteins, and dairy products. These provide essential vitamins and minerals vital for fetal development.

2. Adequate Caloric Intake:
While "eating for two" is a common saying, it doesn't mean doubling your calorie intake. Instead, opt for an

additional 300-500 calories daily, emphasizing quality over quantity.

3. Protein Power:

Protein is a key player in pregnancy nutrition. Include sources like lean meat, poultry, fish, eggs, legumes, and dairy to support the baby's growth and repair maternal tissues.

4. Essential Fats:

Incorporate healthy fats, such as omega-3 fatty acids found in fish, flaxseeds, and walnuts. These contribute to the baby's brain and eye development.

5. Iron and Calcium:

Ensure an adequate intake of iron and calcium. Iron-rich foods like spinach and lean meats prevent anemia, while dairy products and fortified foods support bone development.

6. Hydration Matters:
Stay well-hydrated. Water aids in digestion, helps prevent constipation, and supports amniotic fluid levels. Aim for at least eight glasses of water daily.

7. Limit Caffeine and Avoid Harmful Substances:
Moderate caffeine intake and avoid alcohol and tobacco. These substances can negatively impact fetal development and pose health risks.

8. Balanced Meals:

Opt for balanced meals with a mix of carbohydrates, proteins, and healthy fats. This helps regulate blood sugar levels, ensuring sustained energy for both mother and baby.

9. Regular Snacking:
Incorporate healthy snacks between meals to keep energy levels stable. Nutritious options include fruits, yogurt, and nuts.

10. Listen to Your Body:
Pay attention to cravings and aversions, but maintain a balance. Cravings may indicate a need for specific nutrients, but moderation is key.

11. Consult with Healthcare Providers:

Regularly consult with healthcare professionals to monitor your nutritional needs and address any concerns. They can provide personalized guidance based on your health and pregnancy progress.

12. Safe Food Handling:

Practice safe food handling to avoid foodborne illnesses that could harm both you and the baby. Cook meats thoroughly, wash fruits and vegetables, and follow hygiene practices in the kitchen.

13. Stay Active:

Incorporate regular, moderate exercise into your routine with your healthcare provider's approval. This helps maintain a healthy weight and promotes overall well-being.

14. Consider Prenatal Supplements:
While a balanced diet is crucial, prenatal supplements may be recommended to fill nutritional gaps. Consult with your healthcare provider to determine the appropriate supplements for your needs.

15. Manage Weight Gain:
Monitor and manage weight gain throughout pregnancy. Aim for a gradual, healthy increase to support the baby's development without excessive strain on your body.

Remember, every pregnancy is unique, and individual needs may vary. Prioritize your health, stay informed, and enjoy this special time while nourishing both yourself and your growing baby.

CHAPTER 3
Essential Nutrients for Mom and Baby

Essential nutrients play a crucial role in supporting the health and well-being of both mothers and their babies during pregnancy. These nutrients are vital for proper fetal development, maternal health, and overall pregnancy outcomes. Let's explore the key nutrients that are essential for the well-being of both mom and baby.

1. Folic Acid:

Folic acid is a B-vitamin crucial for preventing neural tube defects in the developing baby's brain and spine. It's recommended for women to start taking folic acid before conception and continue during the early stages of pregnancy.

2. Iron:

Iron is essential for preventing anemia in pregnant women, ensuring an adequate oxygen supply to the developing fetus. Good sources of iron include lean meats, beans, and fortified cereals.

3. Calcium:

Calcium is vital for the development of the baby's bones and teeth. It also helps maintain the mother's bone health. Dairy products, leafy greens, and fortified plant-based milk are excellent sources of calcium.

4. Omega-3 Fatty Acids:

Omega-3 fatty acids, particularly DHA (docosahexaenoic acid), are crucial for the baby's brain and eye development. Fatty fish like salmon, walnuts, and flaxseeds are rich sources.

5. Vitamin D:

Vitamin D is essential for calcium absorption, aiding in the development of the baby's bones and teeth. Sun exposure and vitamin D-rich foods like fortified dairy products contribute to sufficient intake.

6. Protein:

Protein is crucial for the development of the baby's tissues and organs. Good sources include lean meats, poultry, eggs, dairy products, and plant-based options like beans and tofu.

7. Iodine:

Iodine is vital for the baby's brain development and the prevention of intellectual disabilities. Iodized salt, dairy products, and seafood are good sources of iodine.

8. Vitamin C:
Vitamin C supports the absorption of iron and boosts the immune system. Citrus fruits, strawberries, and bell peppers are excellent sources of vitamin C.

9. Vitamin A:
Vitamin A is essential for the baby's vision, immune system, and cell growth. However, excessive intake can be harmful, so it's crucial to get it from sources like sweet potatoes, carrots, and spinach in moderation.

10. Zinc:

Zinc is vital for cell division and contributes to the baby's growth and development. Meat, dairy products, nuts, and legumes are good sources of zinc.

Ensuring a well-balanced and nutrient-dense diet is fundamental during pregnancy. Additionally, prenatal supplements may be recommended to cover any potential gaps in nutrition. It's essential for expectant mothers to consult with healthcare professionals to create an individualized plan that meets their specific needs.

In summary, providing the right nutrients during pregnancy is essential for the health and development of both mother and baby. A diverse and balanced diet, along with appropriate supplements, can contribute to a positive pregnancy experience and lay the foundation for a healthy future.

CHAPTER 4
Building Blocks: Proteins and Their Importance

Proteins are essential building blocks for life, playing a crucial role in various biological processes. These molecules are composed of amino acids, which are organic compounds containing carbon, hydrogen, nitrogen, oxygen, and sometimes sulfur. The unique sequence of amino acids determines the structure and function of each protein.

The primary functions of proteins are diverse and indispensable. One of their key roles is serving as enzymes, catalysts that facilitate biochemical reactions within cells. Enzymes are crucial for metabolism, enabling cells to perform tasks like breaking down nutrients or building complex molecules. Without proteins, these vital processes would be severely impaired.

Additionally, proteins contribute to the structure and support of cells and tissues. Collagen, for instance, is a protein that provides strength and elasticity to skin, tendons, and connective tissues. Actin and myosin, two other proteins, are essential for muscle contraction, enabling movement and mobility.

Proteins also function as messengers in cell communication. Hormones like insulin are proteins that regulate blood sugar levels, influencing various physiological processes. Antibodies, another type of protein, play a pivotal role in the immune system by recognizing and neutralizing harmful pathogens.

The human body requires a variety of proteins, each with its own unique structure and function. Essential amino acids, which cannot be synthesized by the body, must be obtained through diet. A well-balanced diet that includes diverse protein sources is crucial for maintaining optimal health.

In summary, proteins are the fundamental building blocks of life, involved in enzymatic reactions, structural support, cell communication, and immune responses. A diverse and balanced diet is essential to ensure the body receives an adequate supply of proteins and essential amino acids, promoting overall health and well-being.

CHAPTER 5

Power of Greens: Incorporating Vegetables

Incorporating vegetables into your diet is a powerful way to enhance your overall health and well-being. These nutrient-packed greens are not just a colorful addition to your plate; they bring a plethora of benefits that contribute to a robust and balanced lifestyle.

Vegetables are rich in vitamins and minerals essential for the proper functioning of the body. From vitamin C in bell peppers to the potassium in spinach, each vegetable offers a unique set of nutrients that supports various bodily functions. Consuming a diverse range of vegetables ensures that your body receives the spectrum of vitamins and minerals it needs for optimal performance.

One of the key advantages of incorporating vegetables is their role in promoting heart health. Leafy greens such as kale and broccoli are high in fiber, which helps lower cholesterol levels and maintain a healthy cardiovascular system. Additionally, vegetables like tomatoes contain lycopene, a powerful antioxidant known for its heart-protective properties.

Weight management is another area where the power of greens shines. Most vegetables are low in calories and high in fiber, making them excellent choices for those aiming to maintain or lose weight. The fiber content helps you feel full for longer, reducing the likelihood of overeating and contributing to a healthier weight.

The power of greens extends beyond physical health; vegetables play a crucial role in supporting mental well-being. Nutrients like folate, found in abundance in leafy greens, are linked to improved cognitive function and mood regulation. Including a variety of vegetables in your diet can contribute to a positive impact on your mental health.

Moreover, vegetables are a natural source of antioxidants, which help combat oxidative stress and inflammation in the body. Chronic inflammation is associated with various health conditions, including heart disease and certain types of cancer. By regularly consuming vegetables with anti-inflammatory properties, such as broccoli and Brussels sprouts, you can contribute to a healthier inflammatory response in your body.

Digestive health is another area where the power of greens comes into play. The fiber in vegetables supports a healthy digestive system by promoting regular bowel movements and preventing constipation. Vegetables also contain prebiotics, which nourish the beneficial bacteria in your gut, contributing to a balanced and thriving microbiome.

Incorporating vegetables into your meals need not be a daunting task. Simple changes, such as adding a side salad to your lunch or including vegetables in your morning omelet, can make a significant difference. Experimenting with different cooking methods, such as roasting, steaming, or stir-frying, can enhance the flavors and textures of vegetables, making them more appealing.

Furthermore, the power of greens extends to their role in disease prevention. The diverse array of phytochemicals found in vegetables has been linked to a reduced risk of chronic diseases, including certain types of cancer. For instance, cruciferous vegetables like cauliflower and broccoli contain compounds that have been associated with cancer-fighting properties.

Educating yourself about the nutritional value of different vegetables empowers you to make informed choices about what you eat. The vibrant colors of vegetables often signify specific nutrients; for example, orange and yellow vegetables are typically rich in vitamin A, while dark leafy greens are excellent sources of iron and calcium.

It's essential to emphasize the importance of variety when it comes to incorporating vegetables into your diet. Different vegetables offer different nutritional profiles, so diversifying your choices ensures that you receive a broad spectrum of health benefits. Consider creating a rainbow on your plate by incorporating vegetables of various colors to maximize the nutritional impact.

In conclusion, the power of greens in incorporating vegetables into your diet cannot be overstated. From promoting heart health and aiding in weight management to supporting mental well-being and disease prevention, vegetables are a cornerstone of a healthy lifestyle. Embracing the diverse array of flavors and nutrients that vegetables provide not only enhances your overall health but also adds vibrancy and vitality to your daily meals. So, next time you plan your meals, remember to harness the power of greens for a healthier and happier you.

CHAPTER 6

Fruits for a Sweet and Nutrient-Rich Pregnancy

Consuming a variety of fruits during pregnancy is not only a delightful way to satisfy sweet cravings but also a crucial step towards ensuring a nutrient-rich diet. The benefits of incorporating fruits into a pregnancy diet are numerous, ranging from essential vitamins and minerals to fiber that aids in digestion. Let's explore the colorful world of fruits and how they contribute to a sweet and healthy pregnancy.

Firstly, fruits are packed with essential vitamins that play a vital role in fetal development. Citrus fruits like oranges, grapefruits, and lemons are abundant sources of vitamin C, crucial for the formation of your baby's skin, blood vessels, and bones. Berries, such as strawberries, blueberries, and raspberries, are rich in antioxidants that protect cells from damage, supporting overall health during pregnancy.

Moreover, the natural sugars found in fruits provide a healthy energy boost, combating fatigue and promoting general well-being. The sugars in fruits are accompanied by fiber, aiding in the prevention of constipation – a common woe during pregnancy. Bananas, apples, and pears are excellent choices for a natural energy lift combined with digestive benefits.

Pregnancy often comes with increased blood volume, and consuming fruits rich in iron is essential for preventing anemia. Dried fruits like apricots and prunes, as well as fresh options like watermelon and kiwi, contribute to the iron intake necessary for both you and your growing baby.

In addition to vitamins and minerals, fruits are a fantastic source of hydration. The high water content in fruits like watermelon, cucumber, and citrus fruits helps maintain fluid balance and supports the amniotic fluid surrounding your baby.

Furthermore, the fiber content in fruits aids in managing gestational diabetes by regulating blood sugar levels. Choosing fruits with a lower glycemic index, such as berries and cherries, can be beneficial for maintaining stable blood sugar throughout pregnancy.

Variety is key when it comes to reaping the full benefits of fruits during pregnancy. Each fruit brings its unique set of nutrients to the table, contributing to the overall health of both the mother and the baby. While enjoying the natural sweetness of fruits, pregnant individuals should also consider the diverse nutritional profiles these fruits offer.

Papaya, for example, is rich in vitamins A and C, aiding in the development of the baby's eyes, skin, and immune system. Mangoes, besides being a tasty treat, provide vitamin A and E, promoting healthy skin and vision. Including fruits like avocados, which are high in healthy fats and folate, supports the baby's neural development.

It's essential to be mindful of food safety during pregnancy. Opt for fresh, thoroughly washed fruits to minimize the risk of foodborne illnesses. Avoid fruits with damaged skin and consider peeling fruits like apples and pears to reduce pesticide exposure.

While fresh fruits are a fantastic choice, incorporating dried fruits into the diet can add convenience and variety. Snacking on dried apricots or raisins provides a concentrated source of nutrients and energy, making it a practical option for busy days.

In conclusion, embracing a diverse array of fruits during pregnancy is a simple yet effective way to enhance both the taste and nutritional value of your diet. From vitamins and minerals to fiber and hydration, fruits contribute significantly to the well-being of both the expecting mother and the growing baby. So, indulge in the natural sweetness of fruits and savor the journey towards a sweet and nutrient-rich pregnancy.

CHAPTER 7
Grains and Whole Foods: Fueling Your Pregnancy

Eating a well-balanced diet during pregnancy is crucial for both the mother's health and the development of the baby. Grains and whole foods play a vital role in providing essential nutrients that support a healthy pregnancy.

Grains are a staple in many diets and are a great source of energy, fiber, and various nutrients. Whole grains, in particular, offer more nutritional benefits compared to refined grains. Brown rice, quinoa, oats, and whole wheat are excellent choices, providing complex carbohydrates that release energy gradually, preventing blood sugar spikes.

During pregnancy, the body's demand for nutrients increases. Whole grains are rich in essential nutrients like folate, iron, and B-vitamins, which are crucial for the development of the baby's neural tube, red blood cells, and overall growth. Including a variety of whole grains in your diet helps ensure a diverse nutrient intake, promoting a healthy pregnancy.

In addition to grains, incorporating a variety of whole foods is essential. Fruits and vegetables offer vitamins, minerals, and antioxidants that support the immune system and help prevent birth defects. Leafy greens, citrus fruits, and berries are particularly rich in folic acid, a key nutrient in preventing neural tube defects.

Protein is another crucial component of a healthy pregnancy diet. Whole foods like lean meats, poultry, fish, beans, and legumes provide the necessary protein for the baby's development. Protein also helps in maintaining the mother's tissue and supporting the growth of the placenta.

Dairy products are a good source of calcium, vital for the development of the baby's bones and teeth. Opt for low-fat or fat-free options to ensure proper calcium intake without excessive saturated fats. If you're lactose intolerant or follow a vegan diet, consider fortified plant-based alternatives like almond or soy milk.

Omega-3 fatty acids, found in fatty fish like salmon and trout, are essential for the development of the baby's brain and eyes. Incorporating these sources of healthy fats into your diet can have lasting benefits for both you and your baby.

Hydration is often overlooked but is crucial during pregnancy. Water plays a vital role in the formation of the amniotic fluid, which surrounds and protects the baby. Staying adequately hydrated also helps prevent constipation, a common issue during pregnancy.

While focusing on incorporating grains and whole foods into your diet, it's equally important to be mindful of what to limit or avoid. High-mercury fish, excessive caffeine, and certain unpasteurized or undercooked foods should be limited to reduce the risk of potential harm to the baby.

In conclusion, a well-balanced diet that includes a variety of grains and whole foods is key to a healthy pregnancy. This approach ensures that you and your baby receive the necessary nutrients for optimal development and well-being. Consult with your healthcare provider for personalized advice based on your specific nutritional needs during pregnancy.

CHAPTER 8
Healthy Fats for Brain Development

Healthy fats play a crucial role in brain development, supporting cognitive function and overall well-being. These essential fats, known as omega-3 and omega-6 fatty acids, are integral components of cell membranes in the brain. They contribute to the formation of nerve cells, help maintain optimal brain structure, and support various cognitive processes.

Omega-3 fatty acids, particularly EPA (eicosapentaenoic acid) and DHA (docosahexaenoic acid), are abundant in fatty fish like salmon, mackerel, and trout. These fats are fundamental for brain health, as DHA makes up a significant portion of the brain's structure. Consuming sufficient omega-3s has been linked to improved cognitive function, memory, and concentration.

Additionally, omega-6 fatty acids, found in nuts, seeds, and vegetable oils, are essential for brain development. Linoleic acid, a type of omega-6, contributes to the synthesis of other important fatty acids that play a role in maintaining brain health.

Including sources of healthy fats in the diet is particularly crucial during pregnancy and early childhood when the brain undergoes rapid development. Pregnant women are often advised to consume omega-3-rich foods to support the fetal brain's growth and development. Breast milk, which is a primary source of nutrition for infants, naturally contains DHA, emphasizing its significance for early brain development.

As children grow, maintaining a diet rich in healthy fats continues to be essential for ongoing brain function. School-age children and adolescents require these nutrients for learning, memory consolidation, and overall cognitive performance. In fact, some studies suggest that a diet deficient in omega-3s may be associated with an increased risk of attention and behavioral issues in children.

Beyond childhood, healthy fats remain crucial for adult brain health. They support cognitive function, memory, and can even play a role in preventing age-related cognitive decline. The brain's high fat content underscores the importance of providing it with the right kinds of fats to ensure optimal performance throughout life.

Incorporating healthy fats into one's diet doesn't have to be complicated. Simple dietary changes can make a significant impact. Including fatty fish in meals a few times a week, incorporating nuts and seeds into snacks, and choosing oils rich in omega-3s and omega-6s for cooking are practical ways to boost healthy fat intake. Additionally, avocados, olive oil, and flaxseeds are versatile options that can easily be integrated into various dishes.

It's important to note that moderation is key, as excessive consumption of any type of fat can have negative health implications. Striking a balance between different types of fats and being mindful of overall calorie intake is crucial for maintaining a healthy lifestyle.

In conclusion, healthy fats are essential for brain development and function at every stage of life. From supporting fetal brain growth during pregnancy to maintaining cognitive health in older adults, these fats play a vital role in ensuring optimal brain performance. By making conscious choices to include omega-3 and omega-6-rich foods in our diets, we can contribute to the overall well-being of our brains and enhance our cognitive abilities throughout life.

CHAPTER 9
Hydration: The Key to a Well-Nourished Pregnancy

Hydration during pregnancy is crucial for the well-being of both the mother and the developing baby. This vital aspect of maternal health often goes unnoticed, yet it plays a fundamental role in ensuring a healthy pregnancy and a positive outcome.

Pregnant women undergo numerous physiological changes, and increased blood volume is one of them. Proper hydration aids in maintaining optimal blood circulation, reducing the risk of complications such as preterm labor and low amniotic fluid levels. Additionally, staying well-hydrated helps alleviate common discomforts like swelling and constipation.

Water is not only essential for the mother's health but also for the baby's growth and development. Adequate hydration supports the amniotic fluid, a vital cushion for the growing fetus. This fluid provides a protective environment, facilitating the baby's movement and lung development. Insufficient hydration can lead to a decrease in amniotic fluid, potentially impacting the baby's overall health.

Furthermore, staying hydrated is integral in preventing urinary tract infections (UTIs) and gestational diabetes, common issues during pregnancy. Proper hydration aids in flushing out toxins from the body and maintaining healthy kidney function, reducing the risk of infections.

For women with gestational diabetes, maintaining stable blood sugar levels is crucial, and hydration contributes to this by supporting the body's natural regulatory processes.

Dehydration during pregnancy can also lead to complications such as overheating, dizziness, and contractions. When the body lacks adequate fluids, it becomes challenging to regulate temperature, potentially causing discomfort and, in severe cases, heat-related complications. Dehydration-induced contractions may trigger preterm labor, posing a risk to both the mother and the baby.

Choosing the right beverages is equally important for pregnant women. While water is the primary source of hydration, other options such as herbal teas and natural fruit juices can contribute to overall fluid intake. Caffeine and sugary drinks should be consumed in moderation, as excessive intake may lead to dehydration and potential adverse effects.

Pregnant women often experience morning sickness, which can contribute to dehydration. To combat this, sipping water throughout the day and consuming hydrating foods like watermelon or cucumber can help maintain fluid balance. Additionally, paying attention to the color of urine can serve as an easy indicator of hydration status – pale yellow indicates proper hydration, while dark yellow may suggest dehydration.

In conclusion, maintaining proper hydration is a cornerstone of a healthy pregnancy. The benefits extend beyond the mother's well-being to include the optimal growth and development of the baby. Adequate fluid intake supports various physiological processes, reducing the risk of complications and promoting a positive pregnancy experience. Prioritizing hydration is a simple yet powerful way for expectant mothers to contribute to a well-nourished and thriving pregnancy.

CHAPTER 10
Managing Cravings and Snacking Smartly

Managing cravings and snacking smartly is crucial for maintaining a healthy lifestyle. It involves making mindful choices, understanding the triggers behind cravings, and finding nutritious alternatives. By adopting a few simple strategies, you can navigate cravings effectively and make snacking a positive aspect of your diet.

One fundamental aspect of managing cravings is to listen to your body. Often, cravings are signals that your body is in need of specific nutrients. Instead of succumbing to unhealthy snacks, try to identify the nutritional deficiencies that might be causing those cravings. If you crave something sweet, it could be an indication that your body needs carbohydrates. Opt for whole grains or fruits to satisfy that craving in a healthier way.

Additionally, staying hydrated is crucial for managing cravings. Sometimes, the body may signal hunger when it's actually thirsty. Drinking a glass of water before reaching for a snack can help determine if the craving is genuine or a result of dehydration.

Understanding the emotional aspect of cravings is also essential. Stress, boredom, or emotions can trigger the desire for certain foods. Developing alternative coping mechanisms, such as taking a short walk, practicing deep breathing, or engaging in a hobby, can help divert the mind from unhealthy snacking.

Creating a structured meal plan with balanced nutrients can contribute to reducing cravings. Ensuring that each meal includes a combination of protein, healthy fats, and carbohydrates helps maintain steady blood sugar levels, preventing sudden spikes and crashes that can lead to cravings.

When it comes to snacking smartly, preparation is key. Stock your pantry and refrigerator with wholesome snacks like nuts, seeds, yogurt, and fresh fruits and vegetables. Having these options readily available makes it easier to make nutritious choices when hunger strikes.

Portion control is another crucial aspect of smart snacking. Even healthy snacks can contribute to excess calorie intake if consumed in large quantities. Use smaller bowls or containers to manage portion sizes and prevent mindless overeating.

Choosing snacks that provide a balance of macronutrients can help keep you satiated for longer. Combining protein, fiber, and healthy fats in your snacks can help curb hunger and prevent the need for frequent snacking.

Mindful eating is a practice that encourages being present and fully engaged with your food. Take the time to savor each bite, appreciating the flavors and textures. This approach can enhance satisfaction and reduce the likelihood of overeating.

Reading nutrition labels is crucial for making informed choices. Be mindful of hidden sugars, excessive sodium, and unhealthy fats in packaged snacks. Opt for whole, minimally processed foods whenever possible, and be aware of the ingredients list to make healthier choices.

It's essential to acknowledge that occasional indulgence is a normal part of a balanced diet. Completely depriving yourself of your favorite treats may lead to cravings becoming more intense. Instead, allow yourself occasional treats in moderation, savoring them without guilt.

In summary, managing cravings and snacking smartly involves listening to your body, understanding emotional triggers, staying hydrated, and making mindful food choices. By incorporating these strategies into your daily routine, you can foster a healthy relationship with food, promote overall well-being, and achieve your nutritional goals.

CHAPTER 11

Meal Planning Made Easy

Meal planning is a crucial aspect of maintaining a healthy and balanced lifestyle. It not only helps you make healthier food choices but also saves time and money. In this guide, we will explore the key steps to make meal planning easy and effective.

Understanding the Importance of Meal Planning

Meal planning is more than just deciding what to eat for the week; it's a strategic approach to ensure you provide your body with the necessary nutrients while managing your time efficiently. By planning your meals in advance, you can avoid last-minute unhealthy food choices and reduce the temptation to order takeout.

1. Set Your Goals:

Begin by defining your meal planning goals. Are you aiming for weight loss, muscle gain, or simply maintaining a balanced diet? Knowing your objectives will help tailor your meal plans to meet your specific needs.

2. Take Inventory:

Before creating your meal plan, assess what ingredients you already have. This prevents unnecessary purchases and ensures you use items before they expire, minimizing food waste.

Practical Steps to Simplify Meal Planning

3. Choose Recipes Wisely:
Select recipes that align with your goals and are realistic for your cooking skill level. Opt for meals with similar ingredients to streamline your shopping list and reduce costs.

4. Create a Weekly Schedule:
Designate specific days for certain types of meals. For example, reserve a day for a quick and easy recipe, another for a more elaborate dish, and a day for leftovers. This structure adds variety to your diet without overwhelming you.

5. Embrace Batch Cooking:

Spend a portion of your weekend preparing batch meals that can be stored for the upcoming week. This not only saves time but also ensures you have nutritious options readily available when you're busy.

Efficient Grocery Shopping Tips

6. Plan Your Shopping List:
Based on your chosen recipes, create a detailed shopping list. Group items by category (e.g., produce, dairy, proteins) to streamline your shopping trip and reduce the chance of forgetting essential items.

7. Stick to Your List:
Avoid impulse purchases by sticking strictly to your shopping list. This not only

saves money but also prevents unhealthy snacks from sneaking into your cart.

Utilizing Technology for Meal Planning

8. Meal Planning Apps:
Take advantage of meal planning apps that offer features like recipe storage, shopping list creation, and nutritional information. These apps can simplify the planning process and keep everything in one place.

9. Online Grocery Shopping:
Consider using online grocery shopping services that allow you to order ingredients from your meal plan directly. This can save time and reduce the

chances of being tempted by unhealthy choices in the store.

Adapting to Dietary Preferences and Restrictions

10. Customize to Your Taste:
Meal planning doesn't mean sacrificing flavor. Tailor your meals to your taste preferences, making it more likely that you'll stick to your plan in the long run.

11. Address Dietary Restrictions:
If you have dietary restrictions or preferences (such as vegetarianism or gluten-free), plan meals that cater to these needs. This ensures your meal plan aligns with your lifestyle.

Overcoming Challenges and Staying Consistent

12. Be Flexible:

Life is unpredictable, and plans may change. Be adaptable and willing to make adjustments to your meal plan if necessary. This prevents frustration and discouragement.

13. Monitor Progress:

Regularly assess how well your meal plan aligns with your goals. Adjust as needed and celebrate your successes, whether they be sticking to your plan for a week or incorporating more nutritious ingredients.

Conclusion

In conclusion, meal planning is a powerful tool for maintaining a healthy lifestyle. By setting goals, creating a structured plan, and utilizing technology, you can make meal planning easy and sustainable. Customizing your plan to your taste and addressing dietary restrictions ensures that your meal plan is not only practical but enjoyable. Overcoming challenges with flexibility and monitoring your progress will help you stay consistent on your journey to a healthier you. Remember, meal planning is not a rigid set of rules but a guideline to support your well-being and make nutrition a seamless part of your daily life.

CHAPTER 12

Special Considerations: Allergies, Restrictions, and More

Special considerations, such as allergies and dietary restrictions, play a crucial role in various aspects of life, from daily activities to social gatherings. Addressing these concerns is essential for creating inclusive environments and ensuring the well-being of individuals with specific needs.

Allergies, in particular, can range from mild inconveniences to severe life-threatening conditions. The prevalence of allergies has increased in recent years, prompting greater awareness and accommodation efforts. In food-related scenarios, restaurants, schools, and event organizers are increasingly recognizing the importance of clearly communicating potential allergens in their offerings.

Understanding the specific allergens that individuals may be sensitive to is vital. Common allergens include nuts, dairy, gluten, shellfish, and soy. However, allergies are highly individualized, and some people may have less common triggers. A comprehensive approach involves providing detailed ingredient information and adopting stringent cross-contamination prevention measures.

Restaurants, for example, can implement practices like separate cooking utensils and designated preparation areas to minimize the risk of cross-contact. Clear menu labeling indicating allergens can empower individuals to make informed choices about their meals. Additionally, staff training on allergy awareness ensures a proactive response to customer inquiries and concerns.

Beyond the culinary realm, allergies extend to environmental factors such as pollen, dust, and animal dander. Understanding these sensitivities is crucial for public spaces, workplaces, and educational institutions. Implementing air filtration systems, maintaining clean environments, and establishing pet-free zones are practical steps to create allergy-friendly spaces.

In healthcare settings, recognizing and addressing patient allergies is fundamental to providing safe and effective care. Electronic medical records and communication tools among healthcare professionals facilitate the sharing of allergy information, reducing the risk of adverse reactions to medications or treatments.

Moreover, dietary restrictions, whether due to health conditions, ethical beliefs, or lifestyle choices, require careful consideration. Vegetarianism and veganism, for instance, have gained prominence, leading to a growing demand for plant-based food options. Restaurants and food services that cater to diverse dietary preferences not only meet customer expectations but also contribute to a more inclusive dining experience.

Similarly, religious dietary restrictions, such as kosher or halal practices, necessitate specialized attention. Food preparation methods, ingredient sourcing, and kitchen protocols must align with these requirements to respect and accommodate individuals adhering to specific cultural and religious guidelines.

In educational settings, awareness of dietary restrictions is crucial for ensuring the well-being of students. Schools must collaborate with parents and guardians to gather information about students' allergies and dietary needs. Implementing clear communication channels between school staff, parents, and students helps create a safe and supportive environment.

Beyond allergies and dietary restrictions, other considerations come into play. Accessibility concerns for individuals with physical disabilities involve providing ramps, elevators, and designated spaces to ensure equal access to facilities. In digital spaces, website and app developers must adhere to accessibility standards to accommodate users with visual or auditory impairments.

Neurodiversity considerations encompass creating environments that embrace individuals with diverse neurological conditions, such as autism or ADHD. Providing sensory-friendly spaces, clear communication strategies, and flexible learning or work arrangements contribute to a more inclusive and supportive atmosphere.

Furthermore, age-related considerations are important, especially in designing public spaces or services. Elderly individuals may require amenities like handrails, seating areas, or larger fonts for readability. Adapting to the needs of different age groups ensures that public spaces remain accessible and comfortable for everyone.

In conclusion, special considerations, including allergies, restrictions, and various other factors, are integral to fostering inclusivity and ensuring the well-being of individuals across different contexts. Whether in culinary practices, healthcare settings, educational institutions, or public spaces, proactive measures and awareness efforts contribute to creating environments that cater to the diverse needs of the population. Recognizing and addressing these considerations not only reflects a commitment to diversity but also enhances the overall quality of life for individuals with specific requirements.

CHAPTER 13

Staying Active for a Healthy Pregnancy

Staying active during pregnancy is crucial for promoting overall well-being and ensuring a healthy pregnancy. Engaging in regular physical activity can offer numerous benefits for both the expectant mother and the developing baby. However, it's essential to approach exercise with caution, considering the unique needs and changes that occur during pregnancy.

Exercise during pregnancy is generally safe and is associated with several advantages, including improved mood, reduced pregnancy discomforts, and enhanced stamina. However, it's imperative to consult with a healthcare professional before starting or continuing any exercise regimen during pregnancy. They can provide personalized guidance based on individual health conditions and pregnancy progress.

One of the primary benefits of staying active during pregnancy is the positive impact on mood and mental well-being. Pregnancy often comes with hormonal fluctuations and emotional changes, and regular exercise can help alleviate stress, anxiety, and depression. The release of endorphins during physical activity contributes to an improved mood and a sense of well-being, which can be particularly beneficial during the emotional rollercoaster that pregnancy can sometimes entail.

Maintaining a healthy weight during pregnancy is another crucial aspect that regular exercise can support. While it's not the time to focus on weight loss, staying within a healthy weight range is essential for both the mother's and the baby's well-being. Exercise helps regulate weight gain, reduce excess fat, and improve overall body composition, contributing to a healthier pregnancy.

Additionally, staying active during pregnancy has been linked to a lower risk of gestational diabetes. Gestational diabetes is a condition that develops during pregnancy and can have implications for both the mother and the baby. Exercise helps regulate blood sugar levels and improves insulin sensitivity, reducing the likelihood of developing gestational diabetes.

One of the most noticeable benefits of staying active during pregnancy is the relief from common pregnancy discomforts. Regular exercise can help alleviate back pain, swelling, and constipation, which are common complaints among pregnant women. Strengthening core muscles and maintaining flexibility through appropriate exercises can contribute to better posture and reduced discomfort.

Pregnancy places unique demands on the cardiovascular system, and staying active helps improve cardiovascular health. Engaging in aerobic exercises, such as walking, swimming, or prenatal yoga, can enhance circulation, reduce the risk of high blood pressure, and promote a healthier heart. A strong cardiovascular system is essential for supporting the increased blood volume and circulation required during pregnancy.

Maintaining proper muscle tone and strength is crucial for supporting the changing body during pregnancy. As the uterus expands and the baby grows, certain muscle groups, especially in the abdomen and back, may be under increased strain. Targeted exercises can help strengthen these areas, reducing the risk of musculoskeletal issues and promoting better overall body function.

While the benefits of staying active during pregnancy are substantial, it's essential to choose activities that are safe and appropriate for each stage of pregnancy. Low-impact exercises such as walking, swimming, and prenatal yoga are generally well-tolerated and can be adapted to individual fitness levels. Avoiding high-impact activities, contact sports, and exercises that involve lying flat on the back after the first trimester is crucial to ensure the safety of both the mother and the baby.

Listening to the body and making modifications as needed is key when engaging in prenatal exercise. Pregnant women should pay attention to how their body responds to different activities, avoid overexertion, and stay hydrated. Incorporating pelvic floor exercises, such as Kegels, can also be beneficial for maintaining pelvic health during and after pregnancy.

In conclusion, staying active during pregnancy is a valuable component of a healthy lifestyle that benefits both the mother and the developing baby. Regular, moderate exercise can positively impact mood, alleviate common discomforts, regulate weight gain, reduce the risk of gestational diabetes, and improve cardiovascular and musculoskeletal health. However, it's crucial to prioritize safety, consult with healthcare professionals, and choose appropriate activities based on individual health conditions. With the right approach, staying active can contribute to a healthier, more comfortable pregnancy and pave the way for a smoother postpartum recovery.

CHAPTER 14

Postpartum Nutrition: Nourishing Your Body After Birth

Postpartum nutrition is crucial for supporting the recovery and well-being of new mothers. After giving birth, a woman's body undergoes significant changes, and proper nutrition plays a key role in replenishing nutrients, promoting healing, and supporting lactation.

One of the primary considerations in postpartum nutrition is meeting the increased energy demands. Pregnancy and childbirth are physically demanding processes, and the body requires additional calories to recover. However, the focus should be on nutrient-dense foods rather than empty calories. Whole grains, lean proteins, fruits, and vegetables provide essential vitamins and minerals that aid in the healing process.

Protein is particularly important postpartum, as it supports tissue repair and helps in the production of breast milk. Including sources of lean protein, such as poultry, fish, eggs, and legumes, can contribute to a well-balanced postpartum diet.

Omega-3 fatty acids, found in fatty fish like salmon and in flaxseeds and chia seeds, are beneficial for both the mother's recovery and the baby's development if breastfeeding. These fatty acids play a role in reducing inflammation, supporting brain health, and contributing to the overall well-being of both mother and child.

Calcium and vitamin D are essential for bone health, especially during the postpartum period when the body may be recovering from calcium depletion. Dairy products, fortified plant-based milk, and leafy greens are good sources of calcium, while spending some time outdoors can help the body produce vitamin D naturally.

Iron is another crucial nutrient postpartum, as blood loss during childbirth can lead to a temporary decrease in iron levels. Iron-rich foods like lean meats, beans, and dark leafy greens can help replenish iron stores and prevent postpartum anemia.

Hydration is often overlooked but is a fundamental aspect of postpartum recovery. Staying well-hydrated is essential for overall health and can aid in milk production for breastfeeding mothers. Water, herbal teas, and broths can contribute to adequate fluid intake.

It's important for postpartum women to listen to their bodies and eat intuitively. Paying attention to hunger and fullness cues, and choosing nutrient-dense snacks, can support energy levels and help regulate mood.

While addressing nutritional needs, it's essential to be mindful of potential allergens if breastfeeding. Some babies may be sensitive to certain foods consumed by the mother, so paying attention to any signs of discomfort in the infant can guide dietary choices.

In addition to focusing on specific nutrients, postpartum nutrition should also address any specific dietary restrictions or recommendations based on the mother's health conditions or any complications during pregnancy and childbirth. Consulting with a healthcare professional or a registered dietitian can provide personalized guidance tailored to individual needs.

Meal planning and preparation become particularly important during the postpartum period when time and energy may be limited. Having nourishing, easily accessible snacks and meals on hand can help new mothers meet their nutritional needs without the added stress of cooking elaborate meals.

Postpartum nutrition isn't only about physical recovery but also about supporting mental and emotional well-being. Hormonal fluctuations, sleep deprivation, and the demands of caring for a newborn can contribute to stress and mood swings. Including foods rich in B vitamins, such as whole grains and leafy greens, can support the nervous system and help regulate mood.

Self-care is a vital component of postpartum recovery, and nutrition is a key aspect of caring for oneself. It's essential for new mothers to prioritize their well-being and nourish their bodies to support the demands of motherhood.

In conclusion, postpartum nutrition plays a crucial role in the recovery and overall well-being of new mothers. Focusing on nutrient-dense foods, staying hydrated, and addressing specific nutritional needs can contribute to a healthy postpartum experience. Consulting with healthcare professionals for personalized guidance and being mindful of both physical and emotional well-being can help mothers navigate the unique challenges of the postpartum period.

CHAPTER 15

Recipes for a Vibrant Pregnancy

Creating a vibrant pregnancy involves a combination of nutritious and delicious recipes that cater to the unique needs of expectant mothers. These recipes focus on essential nutrients, ensuring a well-rounded diet that supports the health of both the mother and the developing baby.

1. Superfood Smoothie Bowl:
Start your day with a nutrient-packed smoothie bowl. Blend together spinach, kale, frozen berries, a banana, Greek yogurt, and a sprinkle of chia seeds. This bowl provides a rich source of folate, iron, calcium, and antioxidants, promoting a healthy pregnancy.

2. Salmon and Quinoa Salad:
Incorporate omega-3 fatty acids into your diet with a salmon and quinoa salad. Grilled salmon not only adds a delicious flavor but also provides essential DHA for fetal brain development. Combine it with quinoa, leafy greens, cherry tomatoes, and a lemon vinaigrette for a wholesome meal.

3. Sweet Potato and Chickpea Curry: Boost your intake of vitamin A with a sweet potato and chickpea curry. Sweet potatoes are a great source of beta-carotene, crucial for fetal development. Combine them with protein-rich chickpeas, spinach, and a blend of pregnancy-friendly spices for a flavorful and nourishing dish.

4. Avocado Toast with Poached Eggs: Avocado is a nutrient powerhouse, packed with healthy fats, folate, and potassium. Top whole-grain toast with mashed avocado and poached eggs for a satisfying and nutritious breakfast. This combination provides essential nutrients for the development of the baby's neural tube.

5. Greek Yogurt Parfait with Berries and Nuts:

Enjoy a calcium-rich snack by layering Greek yogurt with fresh berries and a sprinkle of nuts. This parfait not only satisfies sweet cravings but also supports bone health and provides a good dose of protein and antioxidants.

6. Quinoa Stuffed Bell Peppers:

Create a colorful and nutrient-dense dinner with quinoa-stuffed bell peppers. Quinoa offers a complete protein source, while bell peppers contribute vitamin C. Fill the peppers with a mix of quinoa, black beans, corn, tomatoes, and spices for a wholesome and satisfying meal.

7. Spinach and Feta Omelette:

Start your morning with a protein-packed spinach and feta omelette. Eggs are an excellent source of choline, essential for brain development. Add spinach and feta for extra flavor and a boost of vitamins and minerals.

8. Chia Seed Pudding with Mango:

For a healthy dessert or snack, indulge in chia seed pudding with mango. Chia seeds are rich in omega-3 fatty acids, fiber, and calcium. Mix them with almond milk and let it sit overnight, then top with fresh mango for a delicious and nutritious treat.

9. Lean Turkey and Vegetable Stir-Fry:

Incorporate lean protein into your diet with a turkey and vegetable stir-fry. Turkey provides iron and zinc, crucial for the baby's growth. Stir-fry a colorful mix of broccoli, bell peppers, carrots, and snap peas for a tasty and nutrient-packed meal.

10. Homemade Trail Mix:
Prepare a nutrient-dense trail mix by combining nuts, seeds, and dried fruits. Almonds and walnuts offer healthy fats, while pumpkin seeds provide iron and zinc. This snack is convenient and provides a quick energy boost while supplying essential nutrients.

Remember to consult with your healthcare provider to ensure these recipes align with your specific dietary needs during pregnancy. Maintaining a varied and balanced diet is key to supporting a vibrant and healthy pregnancy journey.

CHAPTER 16

Frequently Asked Questions

commonly known as FAQs, play a crucial role in providing concise and helpful information to users. These sections serve as a valuable resource, addressing common queries and enhancing user experience. Here, we explore the significance of FAQs, their structure, and some best practices in crafting them.

FAQs serve as a preemptive measure, anticipating users' questions and providing answers in advance. This not only saves users time but also reduces the burden on customer support teams. By addressing common concerns, FAQs contribute to a smoother user journey and can lead to increased satisfaction.

Organizing FAQs effectively is essential. Categorizing questions by topic ensures that users can quickly find relevant information. This logical structure streamlines the user experience, preventing frustration and promoting engagement. Additionally, incorporating a search function within the FAQs can further enhance accessibility.

When crafting FAQs, clarity and simplicity are paramount. Use plain language and avoid technical jargon whenever possible. Users should easily comprehend the information, making the FAQs an inclusive resource for individuals with varying levels of expertise.

Regularly updating FAQs is crucial to maintaining relevance. As products, services, or policies evolve, the FAQs must reflect these changes. Outdated information can lead to confusion and erode trust. Keeping FAQs current demonstrates a commitment to transparency and customer care.

In terms of length, each FAQ should be concise while providing comprehensive answers. Users generally prefer to scan for information, so use bulleted lists or short paragraphs. A balance between brevity and completeness ensures that users quickly find the information they seek without being overwhelmed.

FAQs should not be static; they should evolve based on user feedback and emerging trends. Monitoring customer inquiries and adjusting the FAQs accordingly can enhance their effectiveness over time. This iterative approach aligns the FAQs with users' evolving needs.

To maximize the impact of FAQs, consider incorporating multimedia elements. Visual aids, such as images or videos, can complement textual information and cater to different learning styles. Interactive elements, such as collapsible sections, can further streamline the user experience.

Prominently featuring FAQs on a website or platform is crucial. Users should easily locate this section, typically through a dedicated page or a visible link in the navigation menu. Highlighting FAQs during onboarding processes or at critical touchpoints can also proactively address potential concerns.

In conclusion, Frequently Asked Questions are a fundamental component of user support and information dissemination. A well-organized, regularly updated, and user-friendly FAQ section can significantly contribute to customer satisfaction and loyalty. By addressing common queries proactively, businesses and organizations demonstrate a commitment to user-centric communication. As technology and user expectations evolve, so too should FAQs, ensuring they remain a relevant and reliable resource for those seeking quick and accurate information.

CHAPTER 17

Conclusion: Embracing a Nutrient-Packed Pregnancy Journey

Embracing a nutrient-packed pregnancy journey is a vital aspect of ensuring both the mother's and baby's well-being. Throughout this exploration, we've delved into the significance of a balanced diet, proper supplementation, and the importance of maintaining a healthy lifestyle during pregnancy.

In conclusion, the journey of a nutrient-packed pregnancy begins with a commitment to providing the body with the essential building blocks for fetal development and maternal health. A well-balanced diet, rich in vitamins, minerals, and other nutrients, forms the cornerstone of this journey. From the early stages of conception to the final trimester, each phase demands attention to specific nutritional needs.

Understanding the role of key nutrients such as folic acid, iron, calcium, and omega-3 fatty acids becomes paramount. Folic acid, for instance, plays a pivotal role in preventing neural tube defects, emphasizing the need for its early inclusion in the diet. Similarly, iron aids in preventing anemia, which is common during pregnancy, ensuring adequate oxygen supply to both the mother and the developing fetus.

Calcium, crucial for bone development, and omega-3 fatty acids, beneficial for brain and eye development, further highlight the diverse nutritional demands of pregnancy. While these nutrients are often obtainable through a well-balanced diet, supplements may be recommended to bridge any potential gaps, emphasizing the importance of personalized healthcare.

The importance of hydration cannot be overstated, as it contributes to amniotic fluid levels, supports nutrient transportation, and helps prevent common pregnancy discomforts. Staying adequately hydrated is a simple yet effective practice that can significantly impact the overall well-being of both the mother and the baby.

Beyond nutrition, maintaining a healthy lifestyle is equally integral. Regular, moderate exercise not only contributes to physical fitness but also aids in mood regulation and can alleviate common pregnancy discomforts. Consulting with healthcare professionals to tailor an exercise routine to individual needs ensures safety and effectiveness.

Adequate sleep is another crucial component of a healthy pregnancy journey. Quality rest supports physical and emotional well-being, contributing to a smoother pregnancy experience. Implementing relaxation techniques, such as prenatal yoga or meditation, can further enhance the overall well-being of expectant mothers.

Moreover, managing stress is imperative during pregnancy. High stress levels can negatively impact both maternal and fetal health. Adopting stress-reduction strategies, such as mindfulness, deep breathing exercises, or seeking support from friends and family, can significantly contribute to a healthier pregnancy journey.

Regular prenatal check-ups with healthcare providers are fundamental in monitoring both maternal and fetal well-being. These appointments provide an opportunity to discuss nutritional needs, address concerns, and ensure that the pregnancy is progressing as expected. Open communication between the expectant mother and healthcare professionals is key to addressing any emerging issues promptly.

Cultivating a supportive environment is equally vital. Partner involvement, family support, and access to reliable information contribute to a positive pregnancy experience. Encouraging open communication and seeking emotional support when needed can alleviate anxiety and enhance the overall well-being of the expectant mother.

In conclusion, embracing a nutrient-packed pregnancy journey requires a holistic approach that encompasses both nutritional and lifestyle considerations. A commitment to a well-balanced diet, proper supplementation when necessary, regular exercise, sufficient sleep, stress management, and supportive relationships collectively contribute to a healthier and more enjoyable pregnancy experience.

As we navigate the complexities of pregnancy, it becomes evident that individualized care is paramount. Every woman's body is unique, and factors such as pre-existing health conditions, age, and lifestyle choices influence the nutritional requirements during pregnancy. Therefore, consulting with healthcare professionals to create a personalized plan ensures that the specific needs of both the mother and the baby are met.

Ultimately, the journey to a nutrient-packed pregnancy is not only about providing optimal conditions for fetal development but also about nurturing the well-being of the expectant mother. By embracing a comprehensive approach that addresses nutritional, physical, and emotional aspects, we pave the way for a healthier, happier, and more fulfilling pregnancy journey.

www.ingramcontent.com/pod-product-compliance
Lightning Source LLC
Chambersburg PA
CBHW062109220526
45471CB00010B/3666